How-To Avoid Readmissions

A Guide for Patients and Families during Hospitalization

Written and Published by
T. C. Oakes MBA and
Claudia Barros MSN RN CCM
7821 North 173rd Avenue
Waddell AZ 85355

For my dad, Jose

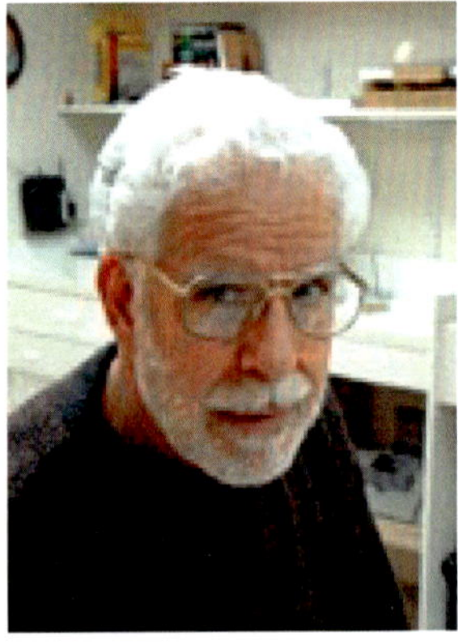

A special thanks to my brother Andre, and my sisters Carmen and Marilia, for asking questions every step of the way and getting our mom safely discharged home from the hospital.

Chapters

Chapter 1
Hospitalization and the Healthcare Team

Admission to the Hospital

When a patient becomes very sick their physician or first responders will send the patient to the nearest hospital. Hospitalization can be a scary and complex process. This book will help patients navigate through the process of hospital admission, develop a safe and understandable discharge plan, and help prevent readmission to the hospital.

Even planned admissions to the hospital, such as surgery, can be stressful. The actual surgery, recovery and the return to work plans can be complicated.

Regardless of whether a patient is admitted to the hospital as an in-patient or placed into observation status, healthcare personnel will want to begin planning for discharge from the very first day of admission.

A well prepared patient and family are vital for a successful and safe discharge home.

The difference between in-patient admission and observation status can often be very confusing. As a general rule of thumb, observation status is assigned based on the diagnosis and the expectation that the patient will be discharged fairly quickly from the hospital.

For example abdominal pain, uncomplicated chest pain, dehydration, lower back pain, nausea and vomiting, pneumonia and dizziness will probably suggest to the admitting physician that the patient should be placed into observation status.

In-patient admission involves staying in the hospital for at least 2 midnights. In-patient admission typically applies when a patient is diagnosed with symptoms of acute heart attack, heart arrhythmias requiring intervention, acute congestive heart failure, acute respiratory failure, and acute stroke with persistent deficits.

Additional diagnoses requiring in-patient status include pneumonia involving 2 or more lobes, bowel obstruction, severe GI bleed, or new onset seizures.

Surgery can be considered either as in-patient or as out-patient admission depending on the complexity of the procedure. Out-patient surgery usually involves same day admission and discharge from the hospital. If complications occur during out-patient surgery, the patient may then be admitted to the hospital as an in-patient for continued monitoring and care.

The emergency room physician along with the hospitalist (i.e. the in hospital physician assigned to the patient) and other specialists will make the determination of admission status based upon presenting signs and symptoms given the insurance guidelines for the admitting diagnosis.

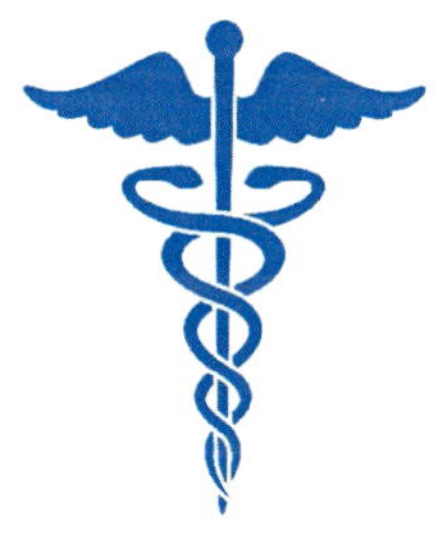

The Healthcare Team

The Healthcare Team consists of physicians, nurses, case managers, ancillary hospital personnel and administrators.

Role of the Physicians

The physician provides continuous care for the patient while in the hospital setting. He or she will examine the patient, take a medical history, diagnose and treat injuries or illnesses. The physician's role includes prescribing medications, ordering tests and procedures, performing surgeries, and interpreting diagnostic tests. The physician has primary responsibility to develop and supervise the patient's overall medical plan of care.

The physicians in the hospital setting include Emergency Room Physicians, Hospitalists or Attending physicians (caring for patients in the Medical Surgical areas), and Intensivists (specializing in providing care in Intensive Care).

Additionally, various Specialists can be consulted when needed to provide proper patient care. These Specialists include:

- Cardiologists
- Pulmonologists
- Gastroenterologists
- Neurologists
- Endocrinologists
- Nephrologists
- Urologists
- Oncologists
- Surgeons

Residents (physicians in training) often participate in the patient's care under the supervision of the Attending Physician or Specialist.

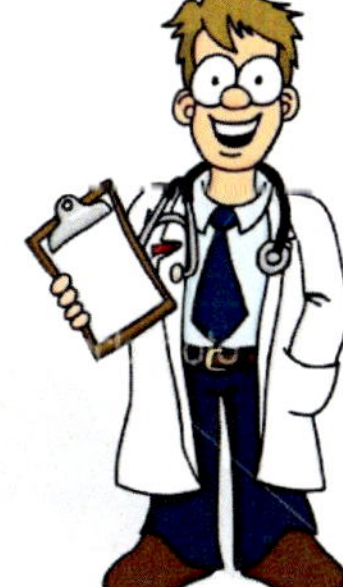

The Physician

Role of the Nurses

The Registered Nurse (RN) has a unique role on the health care team. The RN is responsible for the ongoing assessment of the patient, evaluating the safety of the medical plan of care before implementation, and monitoring the patient's response to the treatment plan.

RN duties in the hospital setting include providing hands-on patient care by administering medications, managing intravenous lines, observing and monitoring the patients' condition, and supervising the care delivered by the nursing assistants.

The RN documents in the medical records and communicates with physicians, patients, families, and ancillary hospital personnel in order to provide the best care possible.

RNs in the hospital setting educate the patient and family regarding the plan of care, new medications, and scheduled procedures. RNs also provide and explain the discharge instructions.

The RN communicates and consults with the physicians involved in the patient's care in order to assure safe continuity of care throughout the patient's hospitalization.

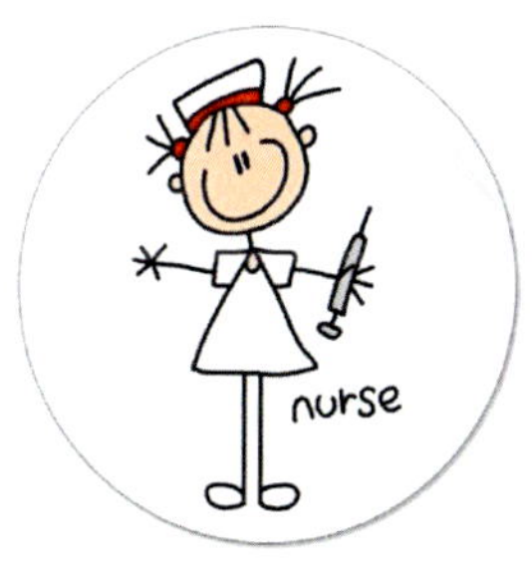

Role of the Case Managers

On the first day of admission, a Registered Nurse (RN) case manager will be assigned to the patient to help the patient and family navigate through hospitalization. The case manager is instrumental in establishing the discharge plan. Other than the physicians and nurses who are treating and caring for the patient, the RN case manager is one of the patient's most valuable resources.

Patients need to be prepared for both hospitalization and discharge. Family members should bring in medications and important health information from home to share with the physicians, nurses and case manager.

The case manager will talk to the patient and family, discuss the case with the physicians and nurses providing care, and review the medical records. He or she will help get answers to any questions or concerns the patient and family may have.

If appropriate, the case manager will make referrals to a Social Worker to assist with discharge needs, or to Patient Financial services if there are any payment or insurance coverage concerns.

The case manager may also refer patients to community services such as the Area Agency on Aging, Patient's Rights organizations, or local community service providers.

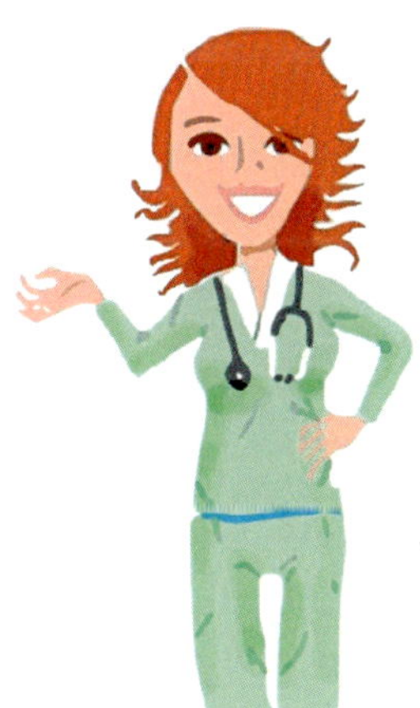

Case Manager

Ancillary Services in the Hospital

The following departments in the hospital will support the physicians, nurses and case managers when providing care. All of the departments work together to assure the care delivery system provides the best possible outcome for each patient.

- Pharmacy
- Laboratory
- Radiology
- Surgery
- Dietary
- Physical, Occupational and Speech Therapies
- Chaplin Services
- Housekeeping
- Maintenance
- Administration

Chapter 2
Insurance and Medicare Plans

Insurance Plans

The patient's insurance plan is specifically designed to provide continuity of care from hospital admission to discharge home. The different levels of care, when properly utilized, can provide the services necessary to prevent readmissions. From admission progressing to lower levels of care, traditional Medicare is intended to help patients improve throughout the process at each level of care as the acuity becomes less and less.

To the extent that other health insurance plans mimic the design of traditional Medicare, the care delivered at each progressive level of care will also help these patients improve their health while reducing the incidence of readmission.

Traditional Medicare, Medicare Advantage and Medigap

Each insurance plan is governed by its own Evidence of Coverage (the Plan Documents). Many Medicare Advantage plans offer similar coverage to traditional Medicare but there will always be variations. The coverage and the cost of coverage can vary. Visit Medicare.gov or call Medicare directly. For patients in a Medicare Advantage plan, call the independent insurance company for specific plan details.

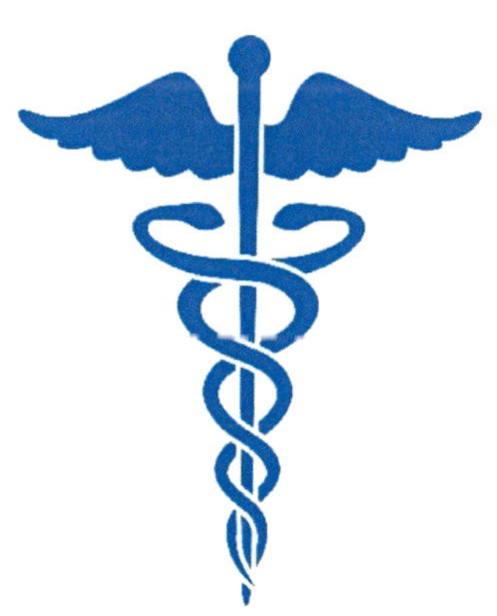

Part A

Part A covers hospitalization. Most patients do not pay a monthly premium for Part A (sometimes called premium-free Part A).

For example, the Part A deductible and coinsurance amounts for 2017 were:

- $1,316 deductible for each benefit period
- Days 1-60: $0 coinsurance for each benefit period
- Days 61-90: $329 coinsurance per day of each benefit period
- Days 91 and beyond: $658 coinsurance per each Lifetime Reserve Day after day 90 for each benefit period (maximum of 60 Lifetime Reserve Days over the patient's lifetime)
- Beyond Lifetime Reserve Days: all costs are borne by the patient

Part B

Part B covers medical services. The standard Part B premium amount changes each year. The premium was $134 (or higher depending on the patient's family income) in 2017. This amount was lower for many patients receiving Social Security benefits (approximately $109 on average), but some paid higher than $134 due to Late Enrollment Penalties.

For example, the Part B annual deductible for 2017 was $183.

If medical services are obtained from medical providers who accept Medicare assignment, traditional Medicare under Part B pays up to a pre-assigned maximum amount per service. In contrast, the patient may be charged more for medical services provided by healthcare providers who do not accept Medicare assignment.

Part D

Part D covers prescription drugs. The Part D monthly premium varies by plan (higher-income patients may pay more). Each Part D plan is administered through an independent insurance company. The plan premiums and pharmacy benefits including drug formularies and coinsurance vary from plan to plan. The overall structure of the deductible is set by traditional Medicare. There was a yearly deductible of $400 in 2017.

The Donut Hole

Most Part D plans have a coverage gap (or Donut Hole). For example, after the patient spent $3,700 in prescription drug coinsurance during 2017, the patient entered the Donut Hole. Once the patient entered this coverage gap, the patient paid 51% of the plan's costs for covered generic drugs and 40% of the plan's cost for covered brand-name drugs until the coverage gap ended.

In 2017, the coverage gap ended when the patient spent a total of $4,950 out-of-pocket. The coverage gap (Donut Hole) will be eliminated at the end of 2020.

Part C Medicare Advantage

The Medicare Advantage plans offered by independent insurance companies through Part C are alternatives to traditional Medicare Parts A and B (and sometimes Part D too). When chosen by the patient during the Medicare enrollment period, Part C replaces Part A and B and sometimes Part D depending on the plan. The Part C monthly premium varies by plan.

Medicare Advantage plans may offer extra coverage such as hearing, vision, dental, gym memberships, and health and wellness. In 2017, many but not all Medicare Advantage plans provided prescription drug coverage that replaced Medicare Part D.

It is important to read the Evidence of Coverage and Annual Notice of Changes when enrolling or re-enrolling in Medicare Advantage plans because the out-of-pocket costs and how the services are delivered (such as physicians, hospitals and networks) vary from plan to plan and can be changed by any plan from year to year.

Many of the services available in Part A, Part B, and Part D (if applicable) are the same as those offered in a specific Part C plan but the costs, restrictions, and pharmacy benefits may vary.

Medigap

Traditional Medicare pays 80% of the Medicare-approved medical expense amounts applicable under Part B. The patient is responsible for the remaining 20% coinsurance. If a patient buys an appropriate Medicare supplemental insurance policy (Medigap plans A-G and M-N) from a private insurer, the Medigap policy will pay this 20% Part B coinsurance amount.

These specific Medigap policies (A-G and M-N) also cover 100% of the coinsurance amounts under Part A, provide up to 365 additional lifetime reserve days under Part A, and cover 100% of the Part A Hospice Care coinsurance.

Medigap Plans B-G and N also pay the hospital deductible under Part A. Medicare Plans C-G and M-N also cover 100% of the coinsurance for Skilled Nursing Facilities. Medigap Plans C and F also cover the Part B deductible.

Medigap policies only work with traditional Medicare Parts A and B, they do not apply to Medicare Advantage Part C nor to Medicare Part D. When selecting a Medigap policy, it is important to evaluate each policy feature given the expected needs of the patient. Select a Medigap policy with policy features that best fit the patient's expected healthcare needs.

Though Medicare has standardized the features of all Medigap policies by providing a capital letter designation for each type of policy, prices vary widely from insurer to insurer offering the same type of Medigap policy. Please shop wisely!

Other Health Plans

There are many health insurance plans offered to patients through employers, unions and the Healthcare Marketplace. Though these plans will include varying premiums, deductibles, coinsurance, covered physician and hospital services, networks, pharmacy benefits, restrictions, and rules, the general structure of these plans will be similar to traditional Medicare and the Medicare Advantage plans.

The patient needs to call the plan sponsor for the specific details of the plan. It is important to read the Evidence of Coverage and other Plan Documents including the Summary of Benefits for the patient's specific plan.

Reading the plan documents will give the patient a good understanding of both the out-of-pocket costs and how the services are delivered for the plan.

Many employers, unions and even some plans available through the Healthcare Marketplace offer separate vision and dental coverage. The patient needs to explore and understand all of their coverage options.

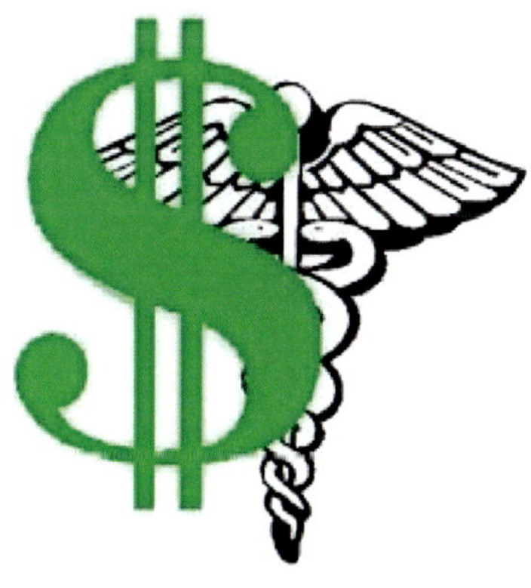

Chapter 3
Traditional Medicare Insurance Coverage

Traditional Medicare Coverage

Traditional Medicare has specific rules regarding which healthcare services are covered. Costs will vary depending on the level of care. Medicare resources at Medicare.gov will provide patients with the most up-to-date information.

Traditional Medicare Benefit Periods

A benefit period is the way that traditional Medicare measures the patient's use of Part A hospital and Skilled Nursing Facility services. Each benefit period ends when the patient has not received any care as a hospital in-patient or in a Skilled Nursing Facility for 60 days in a row.

The Part A coinsurance per day for each benefit period increases the longer the patient stays in a facility. These facilities include in-patient hospital, Acute In-patient Rehabilitation, Long-term Care Hospital, and Skilled Nursing Facility.

In-patient Hospital Stay

- Patient must be admitted as in-patient per physician's orders to be considered in-patient for traditional Medicare coverage purposes.
- Readmission for the same diagnosis within three days of discharge constitutes a continuation of the initial stay.
- Traditional Medicare covers up to 90 days in a hospital per benefit period and offers up to an additional 60 days of coverage with a high coinsurance amount. These additional days are known as Medicare Lifetime Reserve Days.
- The 60 Lifetime Reserve Days can be used only once during the patient's lifetime but do not have to be applied towards the same hospital stay. The Medicare Lifetime Reserve Days only apply to in-patient hospital care.

- If the patient is in the hospital for more than 90 days in a single benefit period, the hospital will start deducting days from the Lifetime Reserve Days.
- For example, if the patient is in the hospital for 95 days in a row, the last five days would be considered Lifetime Reserve Days. The patient would then have 55 Lifetime Reserve Days available for future use.
- The patient may choose anytime to not use their Lifetime Reserve Days and pay the daily coinsurance amounts out of their own pocket.
- For example, if the patient's daily hospital costs are only slightly higher than the coinsurance amount for the Lifetime Reserve Days, then the patient may choose to preserve their Lifetime Reserve Days for future hospital stays that may be more expensive (e.g. Medical Surgical versus Intensive Care admissions).

- The patient pays all of the cost for each day after the 60 Lifetime Reserve Days are used up.

Observation Status

- Staying overnight in the hospital does not necessarily mean the patient is in-patient. The patient is only in-patient if the hospital formally admits the patient and the physician explicitly orders that the patient be admitted as in-patient.
- If the patient is admitted to observation status, they are not considered in-patient even if they are in the hospital for longer than 3 days.
- When in observation status, there has to be a formal physician order for in-patient admission and a formal in-patient admitting process by the hospital before the patient is considered in-patient for Medicare insurance purposes.

- The physician must be able to support and document the in-patient admission orders with a medically-necessary and appropriate in-patient diagnosis.

- It is important to recognize that being considered in-patient or out-patient affects what the patient will pay and determines whether the patient will qualify for Part A coverage in a Skilled Nursing Facility.

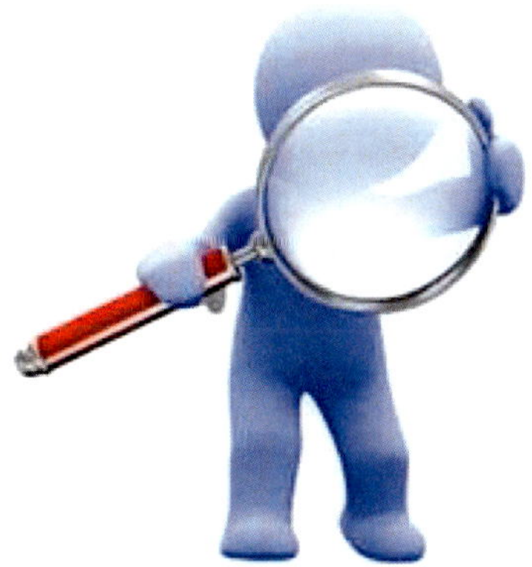

Skilled Nursing Facility

- Part A coverage will only cover Skilled Nursing Facility care after a qualifying 3-day minimum in-patient hospital stay which is considered medically-necessary for a specific illness or injury.

- The in-patient hospital stay begins on the day the hospital admits the patient to in-patient status but does not include the day of discharge. To be considered a qualifying in-patient stay, the physician must specifically order in-patient admission.

- The care provided at a Skilled Nursing Facility must be reasonable and necessary care.

- Traditional Medicare covers up to 100 days of Skilled Nursing Facility care per benefit period.

- A coinsurance amount applies to each day after 20 days in a Skilled Nursing Facility.

- For each spell of illness, traditional Medicare will cover care in a Skilled Nursing Facility only if the physician continues to prescribe medically-necessary skilled nursing care or therapies.

- The physician will need to document expected improvement or the care will be considered Custodial and not covered by traditional Medicare.

- Patient must be out of Skilled Nursing Facility for 60 consecutive days before the benefit period restarts.

- Skilled Nursing Facility care is only covered by traditional Medicare if the Skilled Nursing Facility is treating a hospital related medical condition or a condition that started in the Skilled Nursing Facility while the Skilled Nursing Facility was treating a hospital related condition.

Custodial Care

Traditional Medicare does not cover Custodial Care. Custodial care includes:

- 24-hour-a-day care at home.
- Meals delivered to the home.
- Homemaker services.
- Personal care.

Home Health Care Services

- The patient must be under the care of a physician, and must be getting services under a plan of care established and reviewed regularly by the physician.
- While receiving home health care services, all physician services require a 20% coinsurance.
- Patient must be home bound. Medicare has strict definitions of home bound.
    - The patient has trouble leaving the home without help because of an illness or injury.
    - The patient normally is unable to leave their home because it is a major effort and leaving the home is not recommended because of the patient's condition.
- Home Health Care agencies must be Medicare certified and the care needs to be ordered by a physician.

- In home health care services include part-time or intermittent skilled nursing care (Home Health Care RN) or home health aide services (Nursing Assistants).
- Traditional Medicare pays 100% of the above in home health care services.
- Up to 8 hours per day and 28 hours per week, part-time or intermittent care only.
- Physical, Occupational and Speech Therapy. Normally these services are covered at 80% under Part B, but they can be covered at 100% when they are medically-necessary and provided on a part-time or intermittent basis in the home health care setting.
- Durable Medical Equipment is covered at 80% after the Part B deductible is satisfied. Coverage for most medical supplies is limited.

Hospice Care

- Hospice coverage is provided under Part A of traditional Medicare. Patients who have elected to substitute a Medicare Advantage plan for traditional Medicare (i.e. Replace Part A and Part B with Part C) can elect to use the Part A hospice benefits under current Medicare rules.

- A physician must certify the patient is terminally ill to qualify for the hospice benefit. Terminally ill is defined as expected to live for 6 months or less.

- The patient's physician must again certify that the patient is only expected to live for 6 more months as the patient approaches the end of their 6 month coverage period or hospice coverage will end.

- Part A Medicare hospice covers most all items related to pain relief and symptom management, required drugs, certain medical equipment, aide and homemaker services, medical and nursing services, and spiritual and grief counseling.

- Coverage under Medicare Part A provides very limited in facility hospice care. Medicare Part A only covers short stays for caregiver respite care or medically-necessary, pain or symptom management that cannot be addressed at home.

- Traditional Medicare or Medicare Advantage will continue to cover the costs of approved medical services unrelated to the patient's terminal condition.

Chapter 4
Hospitalization and Patient Responsibilities

During Hospitalization

The patient and/ or family member should keep track of everything that occurs while the patient is in the hospital. Summarize all of the care received in a notebook, any information the case manager or nurses provide, and any discussions with the physicians involved in providing care and treatment.

This information will be helpful in numerous ways. It will allow for review of what has occurred, provide a record for future reference, and enable the patient or family to ask questions of the healthcare team. Patients and families will be better equipped to understand the ongoing medical issues and the care being provided.

Active participation in the care received and in the decisions being made is critical to positive outcomes in a hospital setting.

Family Responsibilities

While the patient is in the hospital, if any family member witnesses anything that seems incorrect … SPEAK UP. The patient's greatest advocate is the family.

Patient's Responsibilities

Encourage the patient to participate actively and in a positive manner in their care. The point of contact for a patient's care is the patient supported by family.

Finding Balance

Accept that once a patient is hospitalized life may be disrupted for possibly a long time. The patient and family members need to find a way to achieve balance, especially when the patient is in the hospital for an extended period of time.

Path to Recovery

The path to recovery involves putting one foot in front of the other, some steps backwards and most steps forward …

Keep taking one day at a time and remembering that some days will be better than others, but every day with your loved ones is a good day.

To do this successfully the patient and family must understand the entire hospitalization process from admission to discharge.

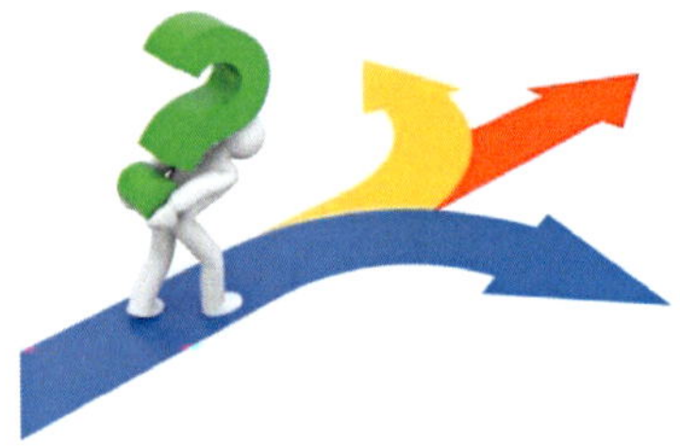

The key to a successful discharge home from the hospital and the prevention of readmission is patient compliance with the medical, nursing and discharge plan of care.

Critical Components of Patient Compliance

- Proper communication between the patient and the healthcare team.
- Accurate understanding by the patient and family of the diagnosis, treatment plan, nursing care, and medications.

- Active participation by the patient and family in the plan of care.
- Diligent monitoring of the patient's care and recovery by the patient, family and the healthcare team.

- Proper utilization of healthcare services.

- Accurate understanding of the patient's insurance benefits.

- Proper assessment and development of the discharge plan.
- Complete understanding by the patient and family of the discharge instructions and home medications.

- Proper patient management at lower level of care facilities.

- Timely physician follow-up after discharge.
- Continuing home care supervision.

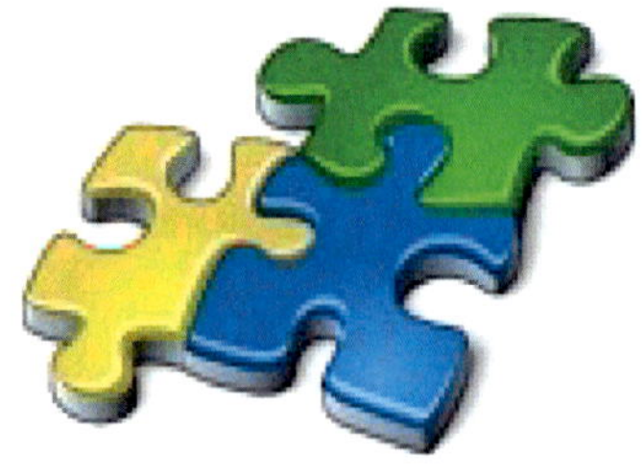

Chapter 5
Managing Hospital Care Information

Introduction

The Hospital Care Summary is a guide to help patients and families summarize the key information regarding the patient's care. The patient or a family member should make notes about the care delivered in the hospital, any treatments provided, and details regarding instructions or teaching the Healthcare Team provides.

Tracking this information will make it easier for the patient and family to better communicate with the physicians, nurses, and case managers. Having the information in a notebook will allow for the patient or family members to review the information and formulate questions to help clarify any concerns and improve understanding.

Hospital Care Summary

The hospital care summary is organized by the key body systems to make communication with the different specialists easier.

Some of the medical issues listed in the hospital care summary can arise during hospitalization or be pre-existing prior to the hospitalization.

Other issues may be related to the patient's diagnosis or to the fact that the patient is in the hospital.

All of these issues should be monitored by the physicians, the nurses, the case managers, the family and the patient.

The better informed the patient is, the more effectively he or she can communicate with the healthcare team.

Communication is an important component of healthcare delivery. Without proper communication with members of the Healthcare Team, the patient and family will have incomplete information when making important healthcare choices.

The hospital care summary will allow the patient to participate actively in the care being delivered and thus return home as quickly and as safely as possible.

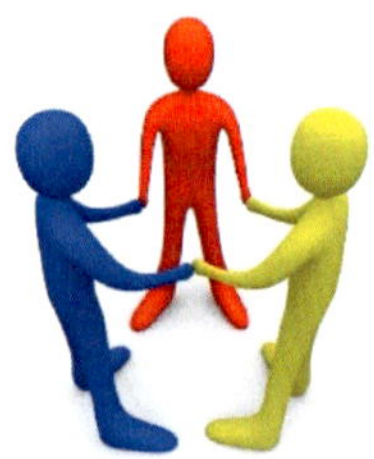

Neurological

Neurologically intact or deficits
Syncope (fainting)
Stroke symptoms
Seizures
Memory issues or Confusion
Fall Risk (safety)
Frequent neurological checks

Gastrointestinal

Constipation and diarrhea
Dehydration
Continuous vomiting
Impaction or bowel obstruction
Swallowing issues and reflux disease
Active bleeding
Need for transfusions
Proper nutrition
Nothing by mouth orders
Nasogastric or feeding tube

Musculoskeletal

Height and weight
Pain management
Intravenous medications for pain
Fractures

Renal (Kidneys)
Bun and Creatinine
Normal urine output of 30 to 60 mL per hour
Avoid urinary tract infections
Intravenous fluids

Pulmonary (Lungs)
Respiratory rate
Arterial Blood Gases
Oxygen Saturation (pulse oximetry)
Oxygen needs
Breathing treatments
Monitor for Shortness of Breath
Prevention of blood clots in the lungs
Normal oxygen saturation is equal to or greater than 94% without supplemental oxygen
Prevention of aspiration and pneumonia

Integumentary (Skin)
Healing of wounds
Avoid bedsores with frequent repositioning and getting out-of-bed as soon as possible
Prevent infections

Endocrine and Laboratory Values

Frequent blood sugar checks

Normal blood sugar range should be 80 to 150

Hg A1C < 7.0

Monitor Hemoglobin and Hematocrit

Monitor INR – maintain 2.0 to 3.0 for patients on Coumadin (warfarin sodium)

Cardiac and Electrolytes

Monitor blood pressure (BP) and Heart Rate (pulse)

Monitor fluid balance for patients with congestive heart failure

Monitor BNP

Cardiac Enzymes (troponin)

Monitor Ejection Fraction (EF)

Monitor electrolytes (sodium. potassium, magnesium, calcium, phosphate and chloride)

Normal potassium is 3.5 to 4.5

Cardiac arrhythmias (such as heart block or sick sinus syndrome)

Nitroglycerin, vasoactive and antiarrhythmic intravenous medications

Infection Control

Hand washing
Proper use of gloves, masks and gowns
High risk for infection due to a debilitated state or bedsores
Temperature (fever) greater than 101.5 degrees Fahrenheit
Elevated White Blood Cell counts
Methicillin resistant staphylococcus aureus (MRSA) or Vancomycin resistant enterococci (VRE) infections
Intravenous antibiotics

Hospital Medications

Monitor narcotic and sedative use (especially in elderly patients)
Insulin use
Heparin use
Diuretics (for fluid overload)

Home Medications Reconciliation

The physicians and nurses in cooperation with the hospital pharmacist will complete a reconciliation of the patient's home medications with any new medications prescribed while in the hospital. Medications that are no longer appropriate will be stopped.

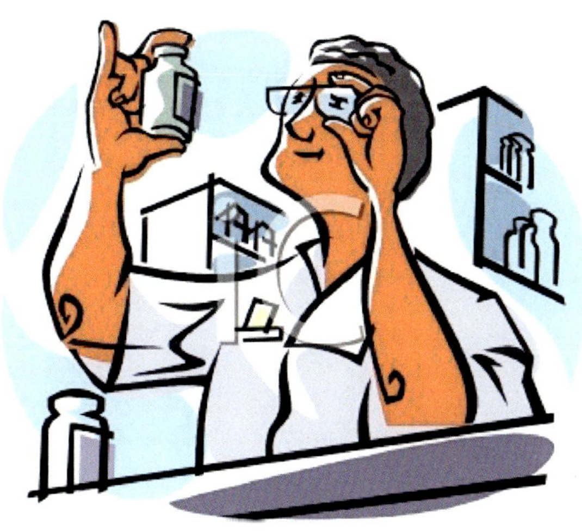

Chapter 6
Keys to a Successful Hospital Stay

Intensive Care

The intensive care setting is an extremely stressful environment for patients and their families. While the patient is critically ill, the case manager, social worker or hospital chaplain can help support the family. The goal of the intensive care physicians (intensivists) and nurses is to support all body systems, stabilize the patient, prevent hospital acquired complications, and avoid antibiotic resistant infections. Once stable, patients will be removed from the ventilator (extubated). Standard medical practice recommends all invasive lines (central lines) and catheters be removed within 3 days. As soon as feasible, patients will be transferred out of intensive care.

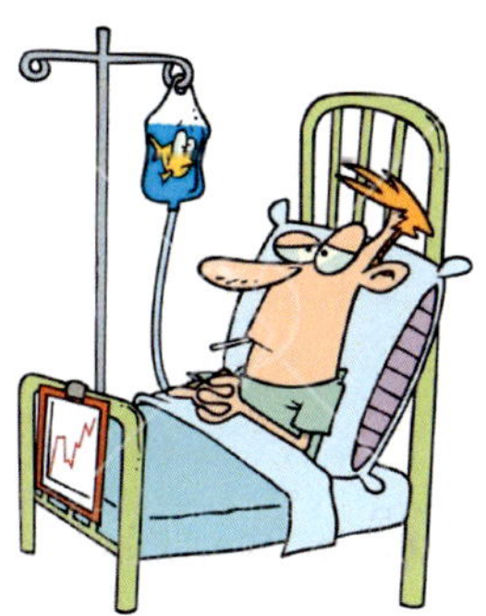

Physical Therapy

Physical, Occupational and Speech therapies will be initiated during hospitalization as soon as the patient is physically able. Make sure the physician orders a Physical Therapy evaluation in order to start the rehabilitation process.

The lack of Physical Therapy may lead to unnecessary complications and can result in prolonged hospital stays. The complications that can occur include atrophy of muscles, loss of strength and lack of motivation, reduced gastric motility leading to constipation and bowel impaction, and the increased risk of blood clot formation.

Procedures Performed

Thoracentesis
Echocardiograms
X-rays (including chest x-rays)
Cat Scans
Magnetic Resonance Imaging
Cardiac Catheterization
Surgeries

Common Medical Errors that can Delay Discharge

Development of a bowel obstruction (ileus)
Bedsores
Development of blood clots

Urinary catheter or central line associated infections
Hospital acquired pneumonia
Aspiration pneumonia
Methicillin resistant staphylococcus aureus (MRSA) or Vancomycin resistant enterococci (VRE) infections

Medication errors such as diuretic, insulin and heparin administration
Overuse of narcotics and sedatives especially in elderly patients
Fluid overload in Congestive Heart Failure patients
Improper monitoring of laboratory values

Delays in treatment
Objects left in the body during surgery
Blood transfusion reactions

Falls with injury requiring treatment
Lack of Physical Therapy

Inconsistencies in communication between members of the healthcare team

Medication Error Example

Insulin administration errors frequently occur in the hospital setting. In one instance, the patient is receiving tube feedings with blood sugar monitoring and insulin administration every 6 hours.

The physician orders the feeding tube be removed in the morning and regular diet to be initiated for breakfast.

At 6am the night nurse administers short-acting insulin as ordered.

At 8am the tube feeding is stopped and the feeding tube is removed. Breakfast arrives 15 minutes later but no one is available to assist the patient with the meal.

The short-acting insulin continues lowering the patient's blood sugar until an astute nurse recognizes the symptoms of hypoglycemia (low blood sugar) and alerts the physician. Treatment is initiated to raise the patient's blood sugar and the nurse assists the patient with a late breakfast.

The risks of insulin administration not followed by food include low blood sugar, seizure, coma and even death.

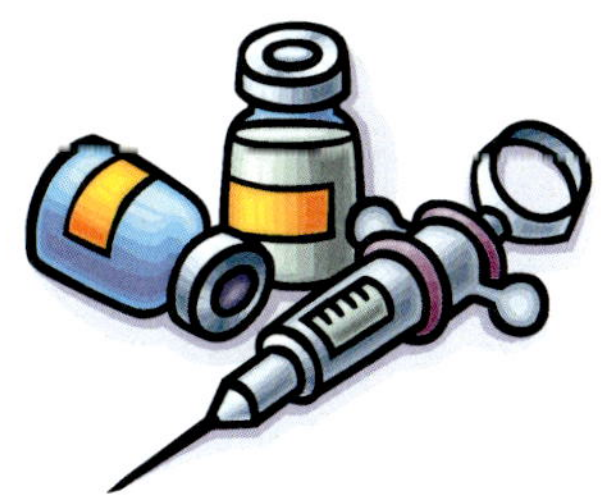

Psychosocial

Stress and anxiety are inevitable factors during hospitalization. Relaxation and stress reduction techniques can be used to help support the patient and family.

Allowing the patient to participate in the decision making process will help reduce stress. It is important to keep patients physically and mentally strong by allowing them to participate in their care as much as possible.

Having family members talk to the patient about non-medical issues will help reduce anxiety. Patients get better sooner with flexible visiting hours.

For patients who are in the hospital for an extended period of time, have family bring in crossword puzzles, music, or books the patient can enjoy.

Wheel chair rides to the lobby or cafeteria can provide a welcome break for patients who are otherwise confined to their hospital room.

If the hospital has a healing garden (with trees and birds) or access to an outside patio, family can check with the physician to see if the patient is allowed to get some fresh air and sunshine.

Nursing can keep the patient and family updated on the plans to go home. All of these activities will help improve their spirit.

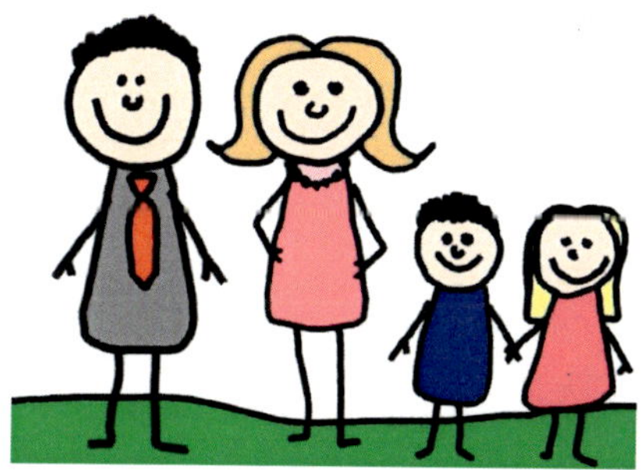

Chapter 7
Care Management Assessment and Discharge Planning

Key Components of the Care Management Assessment

The Healthcare Team will inquire about all of the patient's needs from the first day of admission in order to begin planning the best and safest discharge for the patient. Some of the areas the Healthcare Team will address include:

Family support – Name and contact phone number
Advanced Directives and Healthcare Powers of Attorney
Do-not-Resuscitate status

Home environment - safety, stairs, ramps.
Ability to perform Activities of Daily Living (ADLs).
How much assistance does the patient require for ADLs - Minimum, Moderate, Full assistance.
Is the patient continent, have a tracheostomy, colostomy, urostomy, or any bed sores?

Does the patient have existing feeding tubes, catheters or IV access (PICC lines or Port-a-caths)?
Are tube feedings or intravenous medications currently being administered at home? What delivery systems are being using for the feedings or medications?

How will the patient get home, who will provide transportation, will the patient need assistance or a voucher to get home?

What types of equipment already exists in the home?
Home Durable Medical Equipment – cane, walker, wheelchair, shower chair, raised toilet seat, grab bars, glucose meter, hospital bed, blood pressure cuff, etc.
Respiratory Equipment – CPAP or Nebulizer (SVN) machines.
Home oxygen with concentrator and portable tanks. Home oxygen is appropriate for patients with congestive heart failure, chronic obstructive pulmonary disease or hypoxia (chronic low oxygenation).

How much oxygen is the patient on at home (Liters per Minute, continuous or as needed with activity)?

Does the patient already have Home Health Care services in place – Registered Nurse, Nursing Assistant, Physical Therapy, Occupational Therapy, or Speech Therapy?
Custodial Caregivers.
Community services.

The case manager will identify if the patient and family have any language, hearing or visual barriers.
Identify ethical, cultural, health beliefs and practices that could influence care options and outcomes.
Literacy of the patient, family, caregivers and support system.

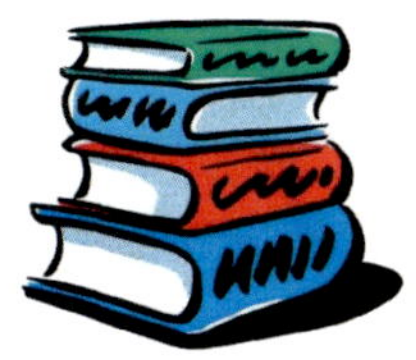

Medical Issues

The physicians will inquire about the patient's current and past medical issues.

Diabetes, cancer, or Wound Care clinic needs.
Any existing infections.
Out-patient Dialysis, the facility name and the weekly schedule.
Does the patient have congestive heart failure, high blood pressure, or a history of heart attack, atrial fibrillation, or chest pain?
Blood clots in the legs or stroke.
History of falls or syncope (fainting).
Chronic obstructive pulmonary disease or pneumonia.
Gastrointestinal bleeding.
Is the patient blind, deaf, or have pain management issues?
Tobacco, drugs or alcohol use.
Are immunizations up-to-date?

Additional Information

The Healthcare Team will verify if the patient has recently been admitted to the hospital. When and for what reasons? Less than 90 days, 30 days or 15 days.

Obtain the name and phone number for the patient's primary care physician and identify if there is an appointment scheduled.
Are there specialists involved in the patient's care? Who are they?
If the patient does not have a Primary Care Physician, the case manager can facilitate finding one.

Pharmacy used and location will be documented. Coumadin clinic for blood thinners. 90-day mail order for prescriptions.
Does the patient have any allergies to medications or otherwise?

What is the patient's ability to pay for medications, equipment or special dietary needs?

Does the patient have benefits such as Veterans Administration, Social Security Disability Insurance, Social Security retirement benefits, Women Infants and Children benefits, or food stamps?

Finally the Healthcare Team will discuss the possible discharge options based on diagnosis and the expected needs once the patient is ready to be discharged.

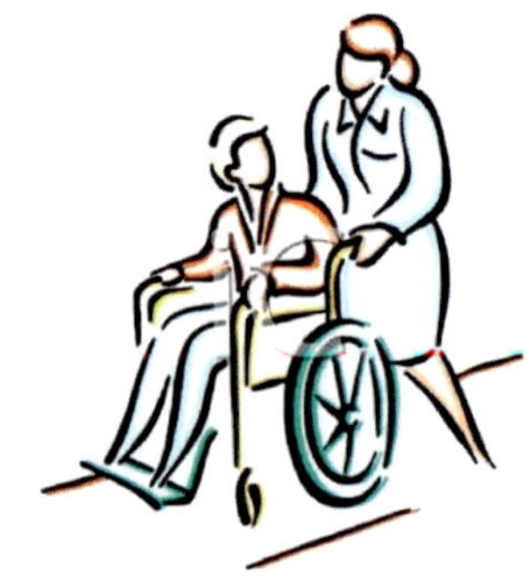

Placement Post Hospitalization

The Healthcare Team will help determine if the patient will need to first go to a Skilled Nursing Facility, Long-term Care Hospital (especially for patients in intensive care), or Acute In-patient Rehabilitation (especially for patients after orthopedic surgery or stroke).

If the patient is unable to return home, will he or she require long-term care in a Group Home setting? Will the patient need a hospice referral?

The case manager will help determine if additional assistance will be needed in the home either from a Home Health Care or Custodial Care agency.

The nurses and case manager will educate, encourage and help arrange the necessary services prior to discharge in order to decrease the chance of readmission and improve the continuity of care the patient receives.

Delays in Transfer to a Lower Level of Care

At times it is appropriate for a facility to delay transfer to a lower level of care (including discharge home) or to transfer the patient to a higher level of care. For example:

Skilled Nursing Facility to Home

The patient has a history of aspiration or swallowing difficulties and vomits excessively on the day the patient is scheduled to discharge home. The Skilled Nursing Facility delays discharge and treats and monitors the patient for another 24 hours.

Hospital to Hospital (higher level of care)

The patient is in the emergency room at a Community Hospital with chest pain and the patient requires emergent intervention only available at another facility.

In other cases, facilities may experience unnecessary delays in transferring the patient to a lower level of care. Frequently, in hospital patients need to be treated for additional conditions, other than their admitting diagnosis, that could otherwise be handled on an out-patient basis. For example:

Hospital to Skilled Nursing Facility

The patient is ready for transfer to a Skilled Nursing Facility but the morning of discharge the potassium level is 3.2 and requires treatment. The physician orders potassium replacement by mouth and a repeat potassium laboratory test 6 hours after administering the potassium.

Delays by pharmacy, nursing or laboratory personnel result in the medication being administered late in the evening and the laboratory test is not obtained until the next morning.

By then, the Skilled Nursing Facility no longer has a bed available which in turn delays the patient's transfer by another few days.

Patients and families should be aware of and monitor for delays that can occur while the patient is in the hospital or in a Skilled Nursing Facility. Unnecessary delays in transfer to a lower level of care (including home) can occur and result in increased medical costs.

Close monitoring for delays and advocating on behalf of the patient by physicians, nurses, case managers, and family members can help avoid unnecessary transfer and discharge delays that ultimately result in higher healthcare expenditures.

Additionally, patients and families have the right to refuse continued unnecessary treatments that only serve to delay discharge especially if the treatments will not positively impact the patient's progression towards recovery and discharge.

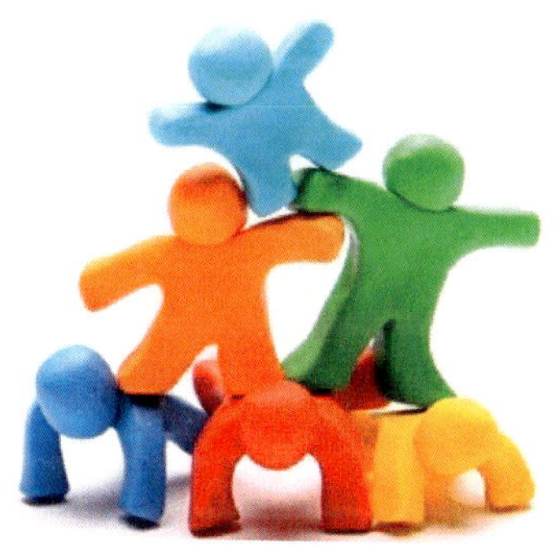

Chapter 8
A Successful Discharge

Planning for a Successful Discharge

Physician Discharge Orders

The physician is responsible for making the decision regarding discharge based upon his or her assessment of the patient's condition.

Once the patient is stable and ready for discharge, the physician will write the discharge orders, complete new prescriptions for all medications, discuss placement plans (Skilled Nursing Facility, Long-term Care Hospital, Acute In-patient Rehabilitation or home) with the case manager, and review discharge instructions with the bedside nurse.

New Treatments Ordered

Orders will be written for any follow-up appointments and treatments needed after discharge (Wound Care, Physical Therapy, Dialysis, and Home Health Care).

Nursing Discharge Instructions

The nursing discharge instructions will encompass the physician orders, new treatments ordered and all medications prescribed for discharge. The discharge nurse will educate the patient and family on the plan of care for a safe discharge home or to another facility if medically necessary.

A Complete Discharge Medication Reconciliation

The physicians and nurses in cooperation with the hospital pharmacist will complete a reconciliation of the patient's home medications and any new medications prescribed while in the hospital. This reconciliation involves reviewing all of the medications previously and currently prescribed and determining the appropriateness of continuing each medication. Any medications that are no longer appropriate will be discontinued.

This reconciliation should be performed regardless of whether the patient will go directly home from the hospital or to a Skilled Nursing Facility, Long-term Care Hospital or Acute In-patient Rehabilitation. All of the current medications and doses will be listed on the discharge medication reconciliation.

Discharge paperwork will include prescriptions for all new medications, including narcotics (30-day supply only) and written instructions for home, Skilled Nursing Facility, Long-term Care Hospital or Acute In-patient Rehabilitation transfer.

Physical and Occupational Therapy Evaluations

Evaluation and treatment plan must be documented within 48 hours of discharge.

Physical Therapy will determine the patient's level of functionality by completing a full evaluation.

A recommendation will be made as to placement (Skilled Nursing Facility, Long-term Care Hospital, Acute In-patient Rehabilitation or Home with Home Health Care if medically necessary) based on the patient's needs.

Criteria used in the evaluation process includes level of assistance needed (Minimum, Moderate or Full assistance), level of independence (stand by to complete independence), bed mobility, ability to transfer, gait (walking requiring what devices) and distance the patient can walk.

When recommending a Skilled Nursing Facility, the Physical Therapist will take into consideration the home situation and family support available. If the patient lives with a capable family member, it may be possible for the patient to be safely discharged home with Home Health Care.

Patients who live alone and have no family support will need to be fairly independent in order to be discharged home safely.

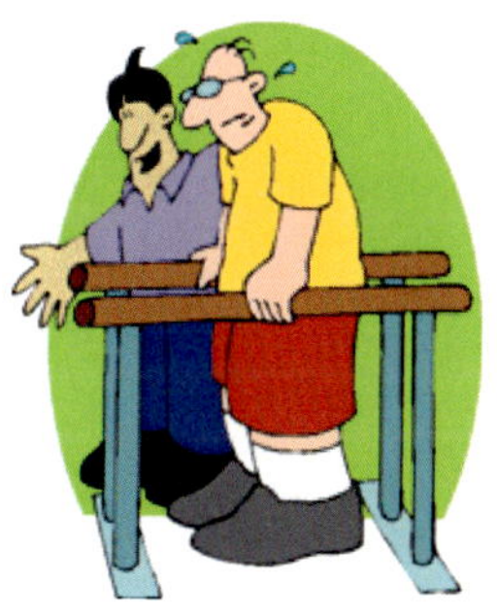

Physician Follow-ups after Discharge (examples)

Primary Care Physician (within 48 hours of discharge)
Surgeon as instructed post-operatively (usually in 2 weeks)
Wound Care (in 1 week)
Specialists - Cardiology, Endocrinology, Pulmonology, Neurology, Nephrology, Urology, Oncology and Gastroenterology (in 5 to 7 days)
Dialysis – Monday, Wednesday, Friday at the specified center and confirmed prior to discharge from the hospital

The patient or family member should schedule a follow-up appointment with the Primary Care Physician before discharge. Call specialist and surgeon offices once the patient arrives home or the next day to schedule additional follow-ups as soon as possible.
Make sure to obtain the Dialysis days and facility information prior to leaving the hospital.

Patient Choice

Once the hospital physician determines the appropriate discharge plan, the case manager will provide the patient with a choice of discharge facilities. Patients can be discharged to a Skilled Nursing Facility, Long-term Care Hospital or Acute In-patient Rehabilitation depending on which criteria they meet.

Acute In-patient Rehabilitation

Criteria for discharge to an Acute In-patient Rehabilitation facility requires the patient be "willing and able" to perform 3 hours of Physical Therapy every day. Patients must also require at least 2 of the 3 therapies offered - Physical, Occupational and Speech. Acute In-patient Rehabilitation patients are expected to make significant functional improvement in a reasonable time period.

Admitting diagnoses for Acute In-patient Rehabilitation typically include Major Joint Replacement, Burns, Brain Injury, Major Multiple Trauma, Femur Fracture, Amputation, Spinal Cord Injury and Stroke.

Long-term Care Hospital

Indications for discharge to a Long-term Care Hospital include Multi-system failure, Ventilator dependence, Complex or extensive wounds, Telemetry monitoring, Complex infections, Chest tubes, long-term intravenous therapy, Total Parenteral Nutrition, Renal Dialysis, complex pain management and patients requiring daily 24 hour physician coverage.

Skilled Nursing Facility

Insurance companies and Medicare only approve admission to a Skilled Nursing Facility if the patient meets certain criteria.

Patients can be discharged to a Skilled Nursing Facility:

- If they have been hospitalized as an in-patient for 3 consecutive midnights or have been hospitalized as an in-patient previously in the last 30 days.

- If they require intravenous fluids or medications, new tube feedings as the primary source of nutrition for this illness, or new tracheostomy for this admission that cannot be managed at home by the patient or family.

- Additionally if the medication prescribed cannot be obtained by the home care pharmacy the patient will be eligible for transfer to a Skilled Nursing Facility.

- For wound care that requires at least once per day dressing changes and daily monitoring by a Registered Nurse.

- When Wound care is less frequent (including wound vacuums) consideration will be given for discharge home. The patient and family will be educated on how to manage the wound with assistance from a Home Health Care agency or Wound Care Clinic.

- Pain Management for a short stay of 3 days.

- Physical Therapy (1 hour per day), Occupational therapy (in conjunction with Physical or Speech therapies), and Speech therapy related to dysphagia and requiring daily monitoring.

- Jackson Pratt drains, T-tubes, ostomies, Pleur-ex and chest tube dressing changes that cannot be managed by Home Health Care agencies and the patient and family.

The case manager will evaluate the patient, family and home situation to determine if the patient's needs can be safely managed and the necessary skills learned in order to discharge the patient home.

Caregivers in a Skilled Nursing Facility are usually Nursing Assistants with RN supervision and Licensed Practical Nurses for medication administration.

Patients will go to a Skilled Nursing Facility in order to regain sufficient function needed for going home. The Healthcare Team can arrange additional services (Home Health Care) for the patient once discharged from the Skilled Nursing Facility to assure a safe discharge home.

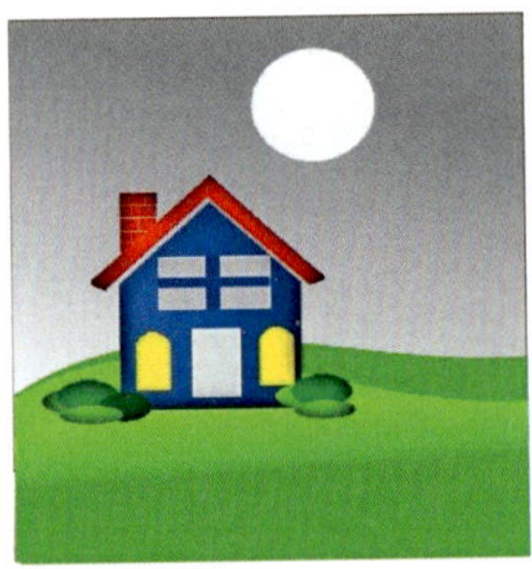

The Move to a Facility

Once the patient and or family have chosen a discharge facility, the transfer of medical records will be handled by the case manager as part of the process of requesting a bed at the Acute In-patient Rehabilitation, Long-term Care Hospital or Skilled Nursing Facility.

Chapter 9
Avoiding Readmission

Readmission Prevention

Once discharged from the hospital, the patient and family should be very diligent in monitoring the patient's condition, care and recovery.

The patient and family should:

- Continue to communicate with the healthcare team after discharge.
- Address any concerns with the physician regarding the treatment plan, nursing care, or medications.
- Actively participate in the patient's plan of care.
- Monitor the patient's condition and report any concerns to the healthcare team.
- Continue to follow the discharge instructions, treatment plan and home medications as prescribed.
- Make sure there is timely follow-up with all physicians involved in the patient's care after discharge.

Sometimes patient's may be readmitted to the hospital for minor issues that could easily be handled at home or in the physician's office, but lack of understanding of the patient's care needs results in the patient returning to the hospital.

For example ... if the patient's blood sugar is a little low in the morning because there was no snack provided the evening before, the patient may be readmitted to the hospital for diabetes management. Instead, the primary care physician or endocrinologist can readily address the need for an evening snack with the family.

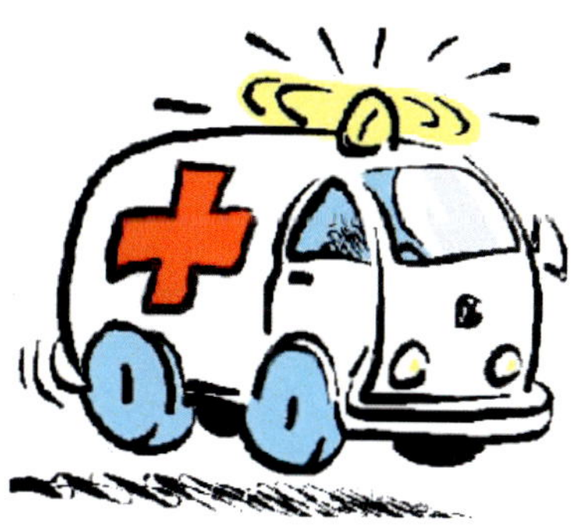

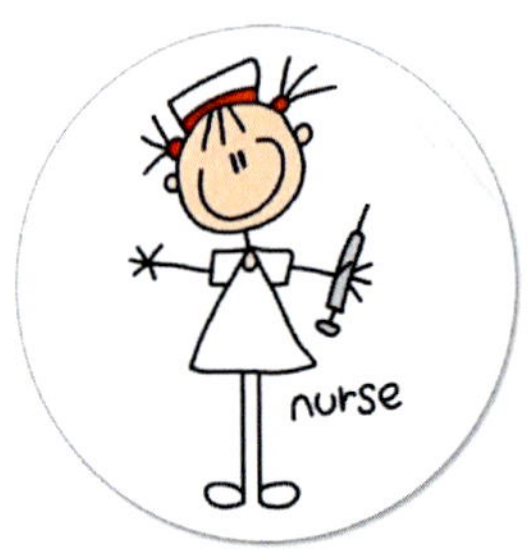

The Nursing Plan of Care at the Facility

The plan of care for the nursing staff at a facility will be determined by the nursing director, charge nurse, the Medical Director, the nutritionist and the Physical Therapy department.

Family should monitor the patient's care, and be directly involved in establishing the Plan of Care. Let the facility know of any special needs the patient may have.

The Plan of Care should include schedules, priorities, best care practices, food, hygiene and Physical Therapy for the patient.

The Plan of Care should also include goals and a time frame for discharge. Make sure the facility is aware of any limitations on Medicare days or insurance coverage. The usual goal for discharge from Acute In-patient Rehabilitation is 7 to 14 days and within 30 days from a Skilled Nursing Facility.

Try to get the BEST accommodations possible for the patient. A quiet, sunny, private room (if possible) will promote healing and recovery. Patients at high risk for infection should not have a roommate. Patients at risk for falls should be in a room close to the nurse's station.

Patient Advocacy

Family should continue to be outspoken every step of the way ... make the patient's needs known and monitor care closely. No one else knows the patient as well or understands the patient's wishes better.

Home with Home Health Care

The Home Health Care RN is responsible for supervising care, medication management, dressing changes and continuing any education that was initiated in the hospital as part of the discharge plan. Nursing Assistants will provide routine care needed to assist the patient with activities of daily living. Physical, Occupational and Speech therapy will come to the home with the goal of transitioning the patient from in-home therapies to an out-patient setting as soon as feasible. In home Physical Therapy is usually scheduled 3 times per week.

Prior to discharge the patient and family should clearly identify when the Home Health Care will start. Remember to obtain the contact information (address, phone number and caregiver name) for the Home Health Care agency.

Home with Custodial Care or Group Homes

An in home Custodial Caregiver is an excellent option for patients who require continuing care post hospitalization but do not meet criteria for a Skilled Nursing Facility.

The caregivers can provide care anywhere from a few hours per day to 24 hours / 7 days per week. The Group Home setting is sometimes more appropriate if the patient requires continuous care or monitoring (fall risk or dementia patients).

Caregivers can be arranged to help the patient with activities of daily living (ADLs) --- mobility, repositioning, hydration, nutrition, medications, hygiene and toileting.

Custodial Care and Group Homes are not covered by health insurance unless the patient has a long-term care policy.

Arranging Home Equipment for Discharge

The case manager will arrange and verify home equipment needs for the patient prior to discharge.

For example --- cane, walker, wheelchair, shower chair, raised toilet seat, grab bars, glucose meter, hospital bed, and blood pressure cuff.
CPAP or Nebulizer (SVN) machines.
Home oxygen with concentrator and portable tanks.
Tube feeding or intravenous medications.
Wound care with frequency and type of dressing changes that need to be continued at home.
Dialysis facility and schedule.
Continuous Passive Motion machine, ice machine or wound vacuum that have been ordered post-operatively by the surgeon.

Home Nutrition

Weight Gain and Healing
6 small meals per day with 300 calories each meal totaling 1800 calories. This will provide adequate nutrition for healing and the strength needed to recover.

As a nutritional guide, follow the Plate Method:
Fill 1/2 of the plate with non-starchy vegetables.
Fill 1/4 of the plate with lean meat (3 ounces cooked) or other high-protein food.
Fill 1/4 of the plate with a starchy vegetable or whole grain serving

Tasty food choices are always a morale booster and appetite stimulant. For patients on restricted diets, the Primary Care Physician will determine when to progress to solid foods.

Home Strengthening

Patients should perform activities of daily living throughout the day. Each activity should be followed by a rest period. Make sure the patient gets 8 to 10 hours of sleep each night with repositioning every 2 hours. Up to chair for breakfast, lunch and dinner.
Varied activity and position changes will help prevent bedsores, promote good circulation, prevent venous stasis, preserve gastric motility and build strength.

Physical and Occupational Therapy 3 times per week. Continue in home exercises daily as well as Occupational and Speech therapies if ordered.

Use of an Incentive Spirometer to help expand the patient's lungs should be continued at home especially for post-operative or post-intensive care patients.

Illness Prevention Strategies

Once the patient goes home, consider setting personal health goals such as eating healthy, losing weight, developing an exercise program, or quitting smoking. Prior to discharge, the case manager, nurses and physicians can help direct the patient on how to plan, set and reach these goals.

Remember ... healthy habits and illness prevention at home will help keep the patient from needing to be readmitted to the hospital.

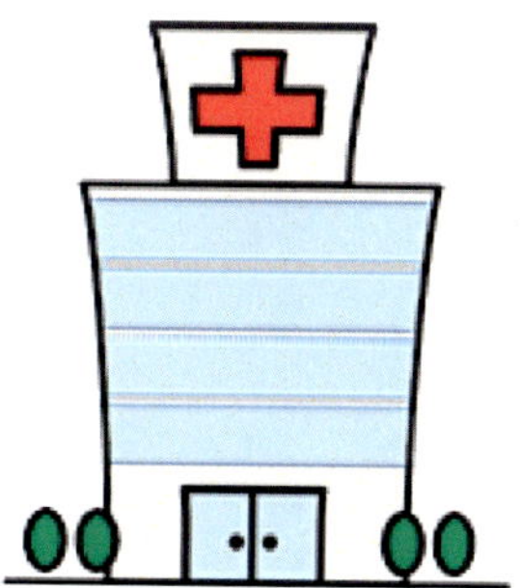

Chapter 10
Tools for Success

Discharge Home Check List (Sample)

- ☐ STAY SAFE --- ASK FOR HELP

- ☐ MEDICATIONS
    - SEE LIST from physician office and SLIDING SCALE for insulin
    - MONITOR for new symptoms or side effects from your medication

- ☐ IMPORTANT LABS AND TESTS (Sample)
    - INR CHECKS
    - MONITOR POTASSIUM
    - BUN and CREATININE
    - HEMOGLOBIN A1C
    - HEMOGLOBIN and HEMATOCRIT
    - BNP
    - EJECTION FRACTION

- ☐ DIET 1800 CALORIES, DIABETIC, LOW SODIUM WITH 2 SNACKS
- ☐ MONITOR BLOOD SUGAR BEFORE MEALS and AT BEDTIME
- ☐ DAILY WEIGHT
- ☐ MONITOR BLOOD PRESSURE
- ☐ CHF MANAGEMENT (Call Primary Care Physician for worsening symptoms)
- ☐ RENAL/ FLUID BALANCE:
  - Sudden weight gain (2 or more pounds in 1 day or 3 to 5 pounds in 1 week)
  - Swollen feet, ankles, legs or abdomen
  - Decrease in how often or how much you have to urinate

- ☐ RESPIRATORY:
  - Shortness of breath or chest congestion which may occur with or without activity
  - Difficulty sleeping except when propped up on 2 or more pillows
  - Frequent dry, hacking cough or wheezing, especially when lying down

- ☐ NEUROLOGICAL:
  - Dizziness, lightheadedness or fainting spells
  - Increased fatigue or the feeling of tiredness

- ☐ CARDIAC;
  - You have tightness or pain in your chest
  - Irregular heart beat / palpitations

- ☐ NURSING CARE:
  - Elevate legs
  - Wear compression stockings

- ☐ CHEST PAIN MANAGEMENT (Angina Pectoris) - Acute Relief
    - 1 tablet under tongue every 5 minutes up to 3 times, use at first sign of chest pain
    - Prompt medical attention needed if no relief, CALL 911
    - Dissolve under tongue, do not rinse mouth or spit for 5 minutes after administration

    - Prophylactic - 1 tablet under tongue 5 to 10 minutes before any activity likely to provoke chest pain

- ☐ PNEUMONIA MANAGEMENT
    - Take vitamin A and C supplement
    - Over the counter cough medication to allow you to rest
    - Drink plenty of water to prevent dehydration

- Avoid people with infections until your pneumonia has resolved
- Wash your hands often
- Cover your mouth while sneezing or coughing
- Hot showers to reduce cough and congestion
- Get plenty of rest to boost your immunity

- Monitor for increased shortness of breath or fever of 101.5 degrees Fahrenheit or greater (NOTIFY PRIMARY CARE PHYSICIAN)
- Stop smoking

☐ WOUND CARE

☐ PT/ OT/ SPEECH IN HOME OR OUT-PATIENT

☐ HOME HEALTH CARE (Start of Care Date) ____________________

- ☐ PRIVATE CAREGIVER HOURS (if needed)

- ☐ HOME EQUIPMENT
  - o CANE
  - o WALKER WITH RAISED PAD
  - o WHEELCHAIR
  - o ANTI-SLIP BATHROOM FLOOR MAT
  - o SHOWER CHAIR
  - o RAISED TOILET SEAT
  - o GRAB BARS
  - o GLUCOSE METER
  - o HOSPITAL BED
  - o BLOOD PRESSURE CUFF
  - o CPAP MACHINE
  - o SVN OR NEBULIZER MACHINE

- ☐ HOME OXYGEN WITH CONCENTRATOR AND PORTABLE TANKS (if appropriate)
- ☐ How much oxygen will you be on at home? Liters per Minute __________, continuous or as needed with activity (circle one).

- PHYSICIAN FOLLOW-UPS
  - PRIMARY CARE PHYSICIAN – Visit scheduled for day of discharge
  - CARDIOLOGY – Call day after discharge for appointment
  - PULMONOLOGY – Call day after discharge for appointment
  - SPECIALISTS – Call 1 to 2 days after discharge for appointment
    - NEUROLOGY
    - ENDOCRINOLOGY
    - NEPHROLOGY
    - UROLOGY
    - GASTROENTEROLOGY
    - ONCOLOGY
    - SURGEONS

Medication Reconciliation (Sample)

The physicians and nurses providing care will complete a reconciliation of all medications before discharge. This will involve reviewing what medications were prescribed in the hospital or Skilled Nursing Facility and comparing them to the medications prescribed for discharge home.

The patient's healthcare providers will determine the appropriateness of continuing each medication. Any medications that are no longer appropriate will be discontinued.

The medication reconciliation should be shared with each physician at the patient's first follow-up visit.

The patient should throw out any old medications that the physicians have not renewed.

SET UP WEEKLY PILL CONTAINERS FOR MORNING AND EVENING MEDICATIONS

TRACK BLOOD SUGAR AND INSULIN DOSES ON A DAILY LOG

Lispro (Humalog) Pen Sliding Scale injection into skin 3 times a day with meals
Check Blood Sugar first @ 7 am 12 noon and 4 pm BEFORE EATING OR ADMINISTERING INSULIN
Eat within 15 minutes of administering insulin
Administer insulin per sliding scale:
150-199 2 units
200-249 4 units
250-299 6 units
300-349 8 units
Greater than 349 10 units
If Blood Sugar less than 60 or greater than 400 --- Call your physician

Lantus Pen 15 units injection into skin at bedtime
Check Blood Sugar first @ 10 pm BEFORE EATING OR ADMINISTERING INSULIN
Administer insulin
Eat a snack

Glucose Test Strips for testing blood sugar

Lancets for testing blood sugar

Metolazone 2.5 mg (diuretic) 1 tablet by mouth every other day

Lasix (furosemide) 40 mg 1 tablet by mouth twice a day

Potassium Chloride ER 20 MEQ 1 tablet by mouth once a day

Omeprazole 20 mg 1 capsule by mouth once a day before breakfast

Nitroglycerin 0.4 mg 1 tablet under tongue every 5 minutes up to 3 times, use at first sign of acute chest pain, call 911 if no relief

Nitroglycerin 0.4 mg 1 tablet under tongue 5 to 10 minutes before any activity likely to provoke chest pain, prophylactic

Levofloxacin 750 mg 1 tablet by mouth every 24 hours

Keppra (Levetiracetam) 500 mg 1 tablet by mouth every 12 hours CLARIFY MEDICATION AND DOSE

Lisinopril 5 mg 1 tablet by mouth once a day

Amiodarone HCL 200 mg 1 tablet by mouth once a day

Coreg (Carvedilol) 3.125 mg 1 tablet mg by mouth twice a day

Coumadin (Warfarin Sodium) 4 mg 1 tablet by mouth once a day

Colace 100 mg (for stool) 1 capsule by mouth twice a day

Silace 60 mg per 15 mL syrup (for stool) 25 mL syrup by mouth twice a day

Senna 8.6 mg (for stool) 2 tablets by mouth once a day

Polyethylene Glycol 3350 (for stool) Mix 17 Grams with 8 ounces water or juice by mouth once a day as needed for constipation

Melatonin 3 mg 2 tablets by mouth at bedtime

Caltrate Calcium 600 mg plus Vitamin D3 800 mg 1 tablet by mouth once a day

Alphagan P 0.1% solution 1 drop in each eye twice a day

Ipratropium Bromide 0.06% Solution 2 sprays in each nostril twice a day as needed

Ketoprophen 20% with 5% Lidocaine (for pain) 1 gel patch on skin twice a day

Tylenol 325 mg 2 tablets every 6 hours as needed for pain

Triad Hydrophilic Wound Dressing apply External to wound every 12 hours

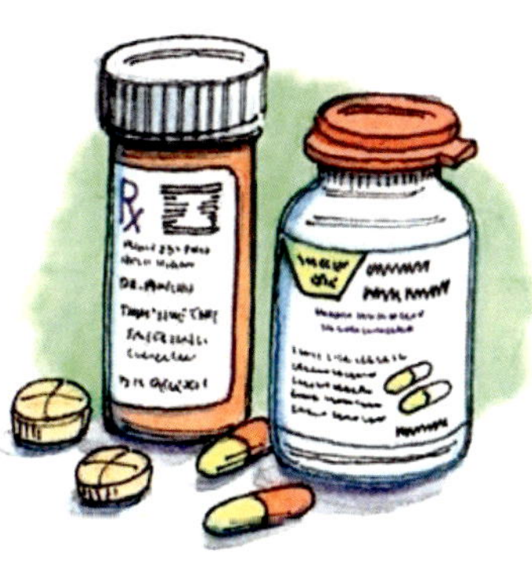

Medications Review Questions to Ask your Physicians (Sample)

Review all of the patient's medications with all of the physicians providing care in order to make sure that the correct medications will be continued.

Review with Primary Care Physician

Insulin and Blood Sugar Monitoring – IMPORTANT TO CONTINUE THESE
Lispro (Humalog) Pen Sliding Scale injection into skin 3 times a day with meals
Lantus Pen 15 units injection into skin at bedtime
Glucose Test Strips for testing blood sugar
Lancets for testing blood sugar

Antibiotic – MAKE SURE THE PATIENT FINISHES ALL OF THIS MEDICATION
Levofloxacin 750 mg 1 tablet by mouth every 24 hours

Stool Softeners, Fiber and Laxatives – DOES THE PATIENT NEED ALL OF THESE? Can the patient substitute fiber in the diet like oatmeal and prunes, a natural lubricant like 1 tablespoon olive oil and fluids including eight 8 ounce glasses of water per day?

Colace 100 mg 1 capsule by mouth twice a day

Silace 60 mg per 15 mL syrup 25 mL syrup by mouth twice a day

Senna 8.6 mg 2 tablets by mouth once a day

Polyethylene Glycol 3350 Mix 17 Grams with 8 ounces water or juice by mouth once a day as needed for constipation

For Indigestion –CONTINUE THIS ONE

Omeprazole 20 mg 1 capsule by mouth once a day before breakfast

For Sleep – CHECK IF THE PATIENT WANTS TO CONTINUE This medication is a very good and natural alternative to sleeping pills.
Melatonin 3 mg 2 tablets by mouth at bedtime

For Pain – IS THE PATCH STILL NEEDED? Once the bedsore heals, Tylenol for occasional aches and pains will probably be sufficient.
Ketoprophen 20% with 5% Lidocaine 1 gel patch on skin twice a day
Tylenol 325 mg 2 tablets every 6 hours as needed for pain

For Osteoporosis –CONTINUE THIS ONE
Caltrate Calcium 600 mg plus Vitamin D3 800 mg 1 tablet by mouth once a day

For Eyes –CONTINUE THIS ONE FOR GLAUCOMA
Alphagan P 0.1% solution 1 drop in each eye twice a day

For Nasal Congestion –CONTINUE THIS ONE DURING ALLERGY SEASON
Ipratropium Bromide 0.06% Solution 2 sprays in each nostril twice a day as needed

For the Bedsore – HAS THAT HEALED?
Triad Hydrophilic Wound Dressing apply External to wound every 12 hours

Review with Cardiologist

Diuretics – DOES THE PATIENT NEED BOTH OR JUST THE LASIX AND POTASSIUM? DOES THE CARDIOLOGIST WANT TO CONSIDER PUTTING THE PATIENT BACK ON THEIR PREVIOUS MEDICATION Triamterene/HCTZ 37.5 mg/ 25mg once a day?
Metolazone 2.5 mg 1 tablet by mouth every other day
Lasix (furosemide) 40 mg 1 tablet by mouth twice a day
Potassium Chloride ER 20 MEQ 1 tablet by mouth once a day

For Blood Pressure, Irregular Heartbeats and Heart Failure – MAKE SURE THE CARDIOLOGIST REVIEWS ALL OF THESE MEDICATIONS AND DECIDES WHICH ONES ARE APPROPRIATE TO CONTINUE. THE PATIENT WAS PREVIOUSLY ON Lozartan Potassium 25 mg once a day.
Lisinopril 5 mg 1 tablet by mouth once a day
Amiodarone HCL 200 mg 1 tablet by mouth once a day
Coreg (Carvedilol) 3.125 mg 1 tablet mg by mouth twice a day

For Chest Pain – MAKE SURE THE PATIENT HAS THIS MEDICATION AVAILABLE AT ALL TIMES
Nitroglycerin 0.4 mg 1 tablet as needed
Follow Chest Pain Protocol

Blood Thinner –CONTINUE THIS ONE
Coumadin (Warfarin Sodium) 4 mg 1 tablet by mouth once a day
Monitor INR as Directed

Review with Neurologist

Anti-seizure - CLARIFY IF THE PATIENT STILL NEEDS TO TAKE THIS MEDICATION AND WHAT IS THE CORRECT DOSE The neurologist started this medication as a preventative for seizures after the patient had brain surgery. Keppra (Levetiracetam) 500 mg 1 tablet by mouth every 12 hours

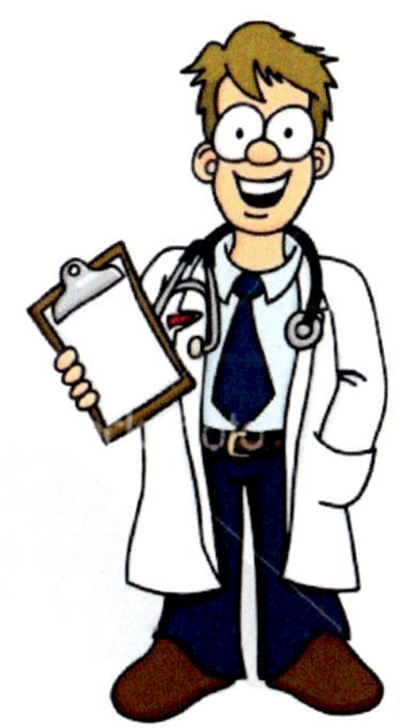

The Physician

The Key to a Successful Discharge from the Hospital and Prevention of Readmission is Patient Compliance.

The Critical Components in Patient Compliance are proper Communication with the Healthcare Team, Patient Understanding of their Benefits and Patient participation in the Plan of Care.

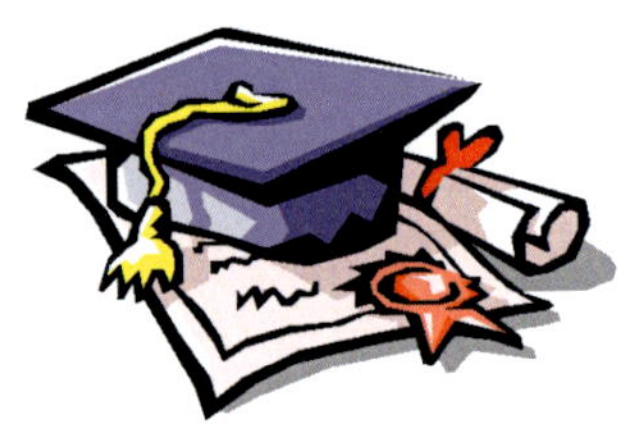

Notes:

Made in the USA
Lexington, KY
16 February 2018